Cecilia Fernández Gil

New studies on Restless Legs Syndrome or Willis-Ekbom Syndrome

Cecilia Fernández Gil

New studies on Restless Legs Syndrome or Willis-Ekbom Syndrome

Imprint

Any brand names and product names mentioned in this book are subject to trademark, brand or patent protection and are trademarks or registered trademarks of their respective holders. The use of brand names, product names, common names, trade names, product descriptions etc. even without a particular marking in this work is in no way to be construed to mean that such names may be regarded as unrestricted in respect of trademark and brand protection legislation and could thus be used by anyone.

Cover image: www.ingimage.com

This book is a translation from the original published under ISBN 978-613-9-05573-9.

Publisher:
Sciencia Scripts
is a trademark of
Dodo Books Indian Ocean Ltd. and OmniScriptum S.R.L publishing group

120 High Road, East Finchley, London, N2 9ED, United Kingdom
Str. Armeneasca 28/1, office 1, Chisinau MD-2012, Republic of Moldova, Europe
Printed at: see last page
ISBN: 978-620-6-27950-1

1. INTRODUCTION

Although Restless Legs Syndrome (RLS) or Willis-Ekbom disease was first comprehensively described in the 1940s, it is only in the last 20 years that it has received greater attention. This has been due to several factors, among which, undoubtedly, its high prevalence in the general population, as well as in some special populations, has played an important role.

Other factors have also contributed, such as the important advances in genetic characterisation, the general impetus provided by the rise of sleep medicine in the developed world, and the potential morbidity factor that this disease represents for other diseases such as cardiovascular or metabolic diseases, not to mention the important advances in treatment. As a result, the number of patients diagnosed and treated for RLS has increased significantly in recent years. Over the last decade, there has been a clear increase in awareness of the disease both in society and in the medical profession. Associations of affected patients have been formed and several drugs have been approved by the health authorities for treatment.

2. DEFINITION

RLS is a sensory and motor disorder that is defined on the basis of four major diagnostic criteria (tables I and II):

- An urge to move the legs, usually accompanied or caused by an unpleasant sensation, pain or discomfort in the legs,

- Symptoms appear and are aggravated in situations of inactivity, such as sitting or lying down,

- Symptoms disappear or improve substantially with movement or stretching of the legs, at least for the duration of the activity, although they may reappear immediately on cessation of movement,

Table I, Diagnostic criteria for Restless Legs Syndrome

- Urgent need to move the legs with sensation of pain or discomfort

- Symptoms appear and worsen with inactivity, sitting or lying down.

- Symptoms disappear or improve with movement

- Circadian rhythm, predominantly in the evening and at nightfall

Table II, Criteria supporting the diagnosis of Restless Legs Syndrome

- Sleep Disorder

- Periodic leg movements during sleep

- Involuntary leg movements during wakefulness

- Normal neurological examination

- Family history,

- Existence of a clear circadian rhythm, with symptoms appearing or worsening in the afternoon and especially in the evening.

The presence of all four criteria simultaneously is necessary to make the diagnosis. However, they are not very specific and not all patients who meet these criteria have RLS.

There are also diagnostic support criteria:

- Sleep disorder.

- Periodic leg movements during sleep.

- Involuntary leg movements during wakefulness.

- Normal neurological examination.

- Family history.

- The compelling need to move the legs is like a compulsion

The urge to move the legs resembles a compulsion, the sensation that precedes a tic. The patient can control it for a while, but the longer he or she goes without moving, the greater the urge to move, while moving the leg brings a temporary relief that is soon replaced by the urge to move again.

Some patients report that if they force themselves not to move their legs, they end up having small involuntary twitches in their feet, especially when they become numb. This need to move their legs is motivated by the search for relief from an unpleasant sensation that the patient feels as something deep, deep inside their legs and which they generally find difficult to define. Some speak of burning, others of bubbling, tightness, pressure ("as if my bones or tendons were being stretched or squeezed"), some call it pain, others simply nervousness, restlessness or uneasiness.

These sensations appear when the patient is at rest, sitting or lying down, and improve with movement. After a variable period of time after sitting, usually a few minutes, but sometimes up to half an hour, the patient begins to feel these sensations. To relieve themselves, they stretch their legs, rub them, wet them with cold water (or more rarely with hot water), until they end up getting up and walking. Walking brings about a very significant and almost immediate relief of the symptoms, but if the patient sits or lies down again, the symptoms reappear.

The disorder has a clear circadian rhythm, at least in the early stages, and patients report that these sensations only occur after dinner or at bedtime.

If insisted upon, many patients admit to having them also in the afternoon, after eating, but generally with much less intensity and with a longer latency between the moment they feel them and the moment they appear.

In general, the worst time is when they go to bed at night with the intention of going to sleep. On the nights of greatest symptomatic intensity (they are not all the same) they are forced to stretch their legs, kick their feet, get up and walk around a bit, unable to sleep even though they are very tired and sleepy. Between 3 a.m. and 5 a.m. the sensations begin to ease and they fall asleep exhausted.

In the morning, when they wake up, they generally do not have these sensations and, if their obligations allow it, they can stay in bed without discomfort.

3. EPIDEMIOLOGY

From Ekbom's early work, RLS was already established as an extremely common pathology, with a prevalence of between 1 and 5%, which was confirmed in epidemiological studies carried out in the 1960s.

However, the lack of uniform diagnostic criteria made it difficult to compare the series studied. The picture changed after the establishment of the criteria set by the IRLSSG in 1995. Several large population-based studies in Europe, Canada and the United States using these criteria found even higher prevalence figures, typically ranging from 5 to 15 % of the population.

However, the adoption of the 2003 revised criteria, more restrictive than those of 1995, gave somewhat lower figures of 4-10%, probably more in line with reality, as the false positive rate decreased.

Racial differences seem to exist and studies in non-Caucasian ethnicities give lower prevalence figures. In Asian countries, most studies find figures ranging from 1 to 4 % of the general population, although others find similar figures to those in the Western population. A study in Africa found a strikingly low prevalence (0.014 %) but significant methodological problems may cast doubt on this figure. Studies looking at prevalence in different ethnicities living in the same place have found a lower prevalence in Turkish, African American or Latin American populations than in Caucasian populations. These ethnic differences are not surprising either, given the importance of genetic factors in the development of this syndrome.

RLS can occur at any age, but the prevalence is higher in later life. Children can be difficult to diagnose and are often diagnosed with other problems, such as attention deficit hyperactivity disorder (ADHD). In all age groups the prevalence in females is higher than in males.

RLS is particularly common in situations that induce iron deficiency or altered iron metabolism, such as pregnancy or advanced chronic renal failure. Approximately 11-30% of women who had no symptoms before pregnancy develop RLS during pregnancy, especially in the third trimester.

4. AETIOLOGY AND PATHOPHYSIOLOGY

From an aetiological point of view, an idiopathic RLS is classically distinguished from forms secondary to various pathologies. Idiopathic forms would be the most frequent, would have a greater genetic component and from the clinical point of view would be characterised by an earlier onset, around 20 years of age. Secondary forms would be related to a causal process and would be resolved when it is resolved. However, as we will see below, this differentiation is not so clear.

Idiopathic restless legs syndrome. Genetic factors

Approximately 65% of patients with idiopathic RLS have a family history and the concordance between monozygotic twins is greater than 80%, reflecting the importance of genetic factors in the aetiology of this condition.

In some families a clear autosomal dominant inheritance pattern can even be established. Linkage studies in these large families with a clear pattern of inheritance have located eight different *loci* associated with the disease, but no single gene mutation has been identified that can cause the disease.

More fruitful have been population studies. Using genomic scanning techniques, which search for polymorphisms, i.e. genetic variants that are not necessarily pathological but can induce changes in the expression or activity of a gene, variants have been identified in four genes (*MEIS1, BTBD9, MAP2K5-LBXCOR1* and *PTPRD*) that increase the risk of suffering this syndrome (table III). These four genes have in common that they are regulatory genes that modify the activity of other genes, some of them related to iron metabolism and transport. Having the polymorphic risk variants does not necessarily mean that one will suffer from the disease, but that the possibility of suffering from it is multiplied by a factor of 3 to 4.

Thus, we are dealing with a disease of a polygenic nature, in the occurrence of which several genes are involved (four known and probably many more that we do not yet know about) with polymorphisms that protect or facilitate the onset of the disease, which will occur as a result of the sum of the effects of all these variants.

Secondary Restless Legs Syndrome - does it really exist?

When reviewing the literature on the aetiology of RLS, it is surprising to note the large number and diversity of disorders that are associated with an increased likelihood of RLS. In these cases it is suggested that RLS may be secondary to these disorders. If we look at them closely, we can distinguish two main groups:

- Circumstances that are associated with impaired iron availability, such as iron deficiency, pregnancy or renal failure, or that cause dopaminergic blockade.

- Processes that can cause pain in the legs, either neuropathic, such as polyneuropathies, especially diabetic, myelopathies or multiple sclerosis, or of another type, such as rheumatoid arthritis or fibromyalgia.

The relationship with the SPI is different in each of the scenarios.

Circumstances associated with impaired iron metabolism or causing dopaminergic blockade

It has already been mentioned that genetic factors are important in the development of RLS and that a genetic predisposition is the breeding ground for symptoms to flourish. On the other hand, we know that there is a link between iron deficiency and RLS as the prevalence of the disease is as high as 30% among individuals with iron deficiency and the intensity of symptoms correlates with the degree of iron deficiency.

We can deduce that, in genetically predisposed individuals, environmental circumstances involving iron deficiency, such as blood loss due to surgery, chronic haemorrhages, frequent blood donations or heavy menstruation, or excessive consumption, such as pregnancy, can unmask or aggravate a previously latent or asymptomatic RLS. Once this iron deficiency has been corrected, RLS may improve and return to the previous situation, but this does not exclude the possibility of it manifesting itself at a later date, perhaps this time without a precipitating factor.

This relationship has been well studied in pregnancy. Approximately one in 4-5 women experience RLS symptoms during pregnancy, especially in the third trimester. This symptomatology usually disappears soon after delivery, but slightly more than half of the women experience it again in subsequent pregnancies. In a follow-up study, 56% of women who had RLS during pregnancy and were asymptomatic after delivery had idiopathic RLS after 7 years and were already chronically ill with RLS.

The same observation is common with other conditions involving iron deficiency or the use of anti-dopaminergic drugs (such as metoclopramide or neuroleptics). Thus, when interviewing patients with RLS, it is not uncommon for them to say that they experienced symptoms after surgery or treatment, that they improved on recovery or discontinuation of the drug, and that they subsequently developed RLS but without the trigger. Therefore, in this case, rather than RLS secondary to iron deficiency or drugs, we should strictly speaking speak of RLS unmasked or aggravated by iron deficiency or drugs. The association of RLS with antidepressant drugs, antihistamines, alcohol, nicotine and caffeine has been described, but the design of these studies is not sufficiently robust to support this causal association.

PATHOPHYSIOLOGY

Since Ekbom's work, we have known that RLS is related to an alteration in iron metabolism. Subsequently, the observation that the symptoms respond to levodopa and that the condition can be triggered or aggravated by anti-dopaminergic drugs led to the conclusion that the pathophysiology of this condition is also influenced by dopaminergic dysfunction. Iron and dopamine are related, as iron acts as a cofactor for tyrosine hydroxylase, which is the limiting enzyme of dopamine synthesis. Moreover, this enzyme is less active in the last hours of the day and iron deficiency further alters its function in the hours of darkness, which could be related to the circadian rhythm that this syndrome follows. On the other hand, in animal models it has been observed that iron deficiency is associated with a decrease in the expression of dopaminergic D2 receptors and the presynaptic striatal dopamine transporter.

RLS results from a dysfunction of the central nervous system. Only dopamine antagonists that cross the blood-brain barrier, such as metoclopramide or neuroleptics, are capable of inducing RLS, while domperidone, which only has a peripheral effect, does not modify this syndrome. Dopamine is a widely distributed neurotransmitter in the central nervous system. The best known dopaminergic pathway is the nigrostriatal pathway, which is affected in Parkinson's disease.

Initial studies using positron emission tomography (PET) and single photon emission computed tomography (SPECT) found no alterations in this pathway in patients with RLS, but other studies have found a deficit or increase in dopamine transporters, and an autopsy study found a lower density of D2 receptors in the putamen in patients with RLS.

The mesolimbic dopaminergic pathway, associated with psychiatric disorders such as schizophrenia, also did not initially appear to be associated with RLS, but a recent study has detected a deficit of D2/D3 receptors in this pathway that correlates with symptom intensity and predicts response to dopaminergic drugs.

Finally, it was observed that destruction of the diencephalospinal dopaminergic diencephalospinal tract (which originates in the hypothalamic area All and terminates in the anterior and posterior horn of the spinal cord), as well as injection of anti-dopaminergic agents into this area in mice, induced the appearance of periodic movements and hyperlocomotive behaviour that mimics what occurs in RLS in humans.

This pathway controls medullary sensory function and has important connections to the hypothalamic suprachiasmatic nucleus, where the biological clock is located and the circadian rhythm is controlled, which could be related to the oscillation of symptoms of this disease throughout the day. In addition, the axons of this system reach the spinal cord, where there are dopaminergic receptors, especially in the lumbar segments. Therefore, it seems to be a good candidate for a link to the pathogenesis of RLS. However, in a necropsy study, no alterations were found in the dopaminergic neurons in this region, but dysfunction of these neurons cannot be ruled out, even if they do not die. Individuals with iron deficiency may suffer from RLS, which is corrected by normalising iron and, above all, ferritin levels. In general, in any circumstance involving reduced iron availability, such as pregnancy or chronic renal failure, the likelihood of RLS is higher than expected in the general population and iron supplementation corrects or improves

RLS symptoms.

However, most patients with RLS have normal or even exceptionally high ferritin levels. What happens is that the onset of RLS does not depend on blood iron levels, but on its availability in the central nervous system. Neuropathological studies with transcranial sonography and magnetic resonance imaging (MRI) have shown a decrease of iron in the substantia nigra and striatum, as well as a low expression of transferrin receptors in these patients, even in those with normal iron and ferritin levels in the blood. This suggests that in RLS there is a problem in the transport of iron to the central nervous system.

In short, everything seems to indicate that in RLS there is a dysfunction in the transport of iron to the central nervous system caused by the coexistence of multiple genetic factors that reduce the efficiency of this transport. If there is a deficit of iron in the blood, transport to the central nervous system, already inefficient, becomes even less effective. But even when blood iron levels are normal, individuals with sufficient genetic load fail to achieve optimal neuronal brain iron levels. Neuronal iron deficiency would cause dopaminergic dysfunction in the A11 area resulting in dysfunction of the medullary sensory pathways and hyperexcitability of the motor pathway leading to the genesis of the periodic motor activity typical of RLS.

A nocturnal disease or a disease with a circadian rhythm

One of the most striking features of RLS is the hourly distribution of symptoms, with onset or aggravation at the end of the day. There is evidence that this oscillation corresponds to a true circadian rhythm of the disease, as the intensity of symptoms correlates negatively with the body temperature curve, and in patients with shift work or trans-oceanic travel, the symptom pattern follows the circadian rhythm, so that it shifts to the time when the individual would be expected to sleep, even if they do not sleep, and gradually adjusts as the individual adapts to the new rhythm.

Presenting a circadian oscillation does not mean that we should consider it as a nocturnal disease. This nuance is not only academic, but is of undoubted practical interest. Although it is clear that symptoms are much more pronounced at the end of the day, patients often have symptomatic flares earlier in the day as well. It is not uncommon for patients to report symptoms after lunch or in the afternoon. But, in general, at these times they are more bearable and the latency from sitting or lying down to onset is longer. However, the predominance of symptoms from 20-21 hours onwards means that therapeutic measures are usually focused on this period of time. Short-term control of the condition may be achieved, but there may be negative repercussions later. The dopaminergic system has a tonic activity and in other diseases with dopaminergic dysfunction such as Parkinson's disease (albeit with a very different pathophysiology to RLS), pulsatile dopaminergic administration is associated with long-term complications. We do not know whether the same is true in RLS, where there is dopaminergic dysfunction and not progressive neurodegeneration as in Parkinson's disease, but a complication of long-term dopaminergic treatment has been described, the "augmentation phenomenon", which is related to the duration of the half-life of dopaminergic drugs. Thus, we should not forget that this is an all-day disease with a circadian oscillation of symptomatology.

5. CLINICAL PICTURE AND SPECIFIC SCALES FOR THE ASSESSMENT OF SYMPTOM SEVERITY

QUADROCLINIC

As we have indicated in the definition, RLS is a sensory and motor disorder in which the sensory component is fundamental and generally the one that motivates the consultation. Patients report a discomfort that is difficult to define, which some call burning, pressure, tingling, tingling, bubbling, pain, etc.

Others simply describe it as nervousness, uneasiness or restlessness. It is mainly located in the legs, between the knee and the ankle, and appears when they are sitting or lying down and prevents them from standing still. To try to alleviate this discomfort, they stretch their legs, rub one against the other, move them and finally have to get up and walk, which relieves the symptoms, although if they sit or lie down again, it soon reappears. If they try to hold still, many notice small semi-voluntary jerks of the legs or feet.

Characteristically, this symptomatology appears more intensely at the end of the day, when they sit down to dinner or after dinner, and especially when they go to bed.

This is when the situation can reach dramatic proportions, as the patient falls asleep, but cannot fall asleep because the discomfort in his legs prevents him from doing so and forces him to move his legs, he gets out of bed looking for coolness and finally has to get up, go to the toilet, walk up and down the corridor or do stretching and walking movements on the spot. Some have an exercise bike in the room. This situation can last until 3, 4, 5 o'clock in the morning, when finally the circadian oscillation allows a decrease in intensity and the patient manages to sleep. And if he manages to fall asleep earlier, he will continue to kick and move his legs periodically even while asleep. In the morning, when he wakes up, he usually has no symptoms, but, even if he would like to, he usually cannot stay in bed, so he is sleep deprived.

Fortunately, in many patients the intensity of the symptoms is variable and not every night the symptoms are so bothersome.

It is therefore clear that there will be a significant impact on the sleep pattern, with an increase in latency and a decrease in sleep efficiency due to the frequency of awakenings. However, curiously, patients do not usually report significant daytime sleepiness, unless they have slept very few hours during the night. The consequences of impaired sleep quality are common to other pathologies in which sleep quality is poor, such as sleep apnoea syndrome, with headaches on waking, anxiety, social isolation, decreased libido and depression. In addition, several epidemiological studies have found a higher frequency of obesity, high blood pressure and cardiovascular mortality in patients with RLS, which could be related to hormonal dysregulation and alteration of the circadian rhythm of blood pressure that leads to sleep fragmentation and poor sleep quality. In addition, each periodic movement has been observed to induce a transient elevation of blood pressure and heart rate.

Symptoms are usually localised in both legs, although they may be asymmetrical and, very rarely, unilateral. In severe cases, other parts of the body are also affected, such as the arms and, more rarely, the belly or face. Exceptionally, they are located exclusively in other regions, such as the genitals or abdomen, without affecting the legs.

Although the disease has an obvious circadian rhythm, it is not uncommon for patients to have daytime symptoms, especially from midday onwards. At this time the intensity of symptoms is usually lower and the latency between the time the patient sits up and the onset of discomfort is longer. The disease usually has a progressive but oscillating course. In the beginning, symptoms appear seasonally, with periods of several months of very little symptomatic duration.

Gradually, however, the disorder tends to become more continuous and of greater intensity, although there are patients who continue to have symptom-free or symptom-free periods throughout their lives.

SPECIFIC CLINICAL SCALES FOR THE ASSESSMENT OF SYMPTOM SEVERITY

IRLS Scale

The IRLS scale measures subjective symptoms of RLS. It was developed by an international group of experts in the late 1990s and has been validated in a large-scale international multicentre study. It is a valid measure of RLS symptom intensity both in those with an established clinical diagnosis and in first-time patients. The IRLS has high internal consistency, inter-rater reliability and test-retest reliability over a period of 1 to 4 weeks, as well as high concurrent validity. It has shown adequate correlation with other generally accepted (although less specific to RLS) severity measurement scales, such as the Clinical Global Impression (CGI).

On the other hand, the IRLS easily discriminates between patient groups and controls.

It consists of ten sections, each of which is scored on a scale of 0 to 4, reflecting the following aspects:

1. Intensity of discomfort in lower and upper limbs.

2. Need for movement.

3. Improvement with movement.

4. Sleep disorders due to RLS.

5. Fatigue and daytime sleepiness due to RLS.

3. Overall assessment of the CPS.

4. Frequency of symptoms.

5. Duration of symptoms over a typical day.

6. Impact of symptoms on daytime activities (family, household chores, work, etc.).

7. Impact of symptoms on mood.

The sum of these items gives a total score ranging from 0 to 40. Subjects with a total score of 0 have no RLS, 1 to 10 have mild RLS, 11 to 20 have moderate RLS, 21 to 30 have severe RLS and 31 to 40 have very severe RLS. Clinical trials testing the efficacy of medicines typically include patients with a score above 15.

The major problem with the IRLS scale is that its score is too dependent on the patient's recall of the last 7 days, does not include any assessment of motor symptoms and does not adjust for physical activity over the days. In clinical studies it has been shown to be very sensitive to the placebo effect.

A clinically significant improvement is considered to exist when the IRLS score decreases by six or more points from baseline.

SPI-6 scale

It consists of six 11-item subscales ranging from 0 ("none") to 10 ("maximum") used to assess the intensity of RLS over the course of a treatment. These subscales are very sensitive for detecting changes in symptomatic intensity during a study designed to quantify response to a drug and to differentiate active treatment from placebo.

The severity of RLS is assessed on the basis of four parameters:

- Intensity of RLS at sleep onset.

- Intensity of the SPI throughout the night.

- RLS intensity during the day at rest.

- Intensity of RLS during the day while performing daytime activities.

6.   DIAGNOSIS

Although the diagnosis of RLS is made on the basis of the clinical criteria outlined above, its insufficient sensitivity and specificity can sometimes lead to both false positives and false negatives. For this reason, in certain cases it is necessary to perform complementary tests as an auxiliary method to ensure the diagnosis and assess the severity.

The diagnostic tests we can use are the following:

■ Laboratory sleep studies:

- Polysomnography.

- Suggested immobilisation test.

- Actimetry.

■ Pharmacological tests.

According to the guidelines developed by the European Restless Legs Sydrome Study Group (EURLESSG), the patient should be assessed by a sleep specialist in the following situations:

1. Poor response to dopaminergic treatment or commonly recommended treatments.

2. Atypical symptomatology.

3. Daytime sleepiness as the main symptom.

Once we have made a diagnosis of RLS in a patient, we have to ask ourselves whether or not to treat the patient with medication.

The decision should be made jointly by the patient and the doctor based on a number of factors. Probably the most important is knowing how RLS affects the patient's quality of life. Thus, we will assess the characteristics of RLS by considering whether the symptoms are sporadic or frequent, their intensity, the time of evolution, the patient's age, whether they occur episodically or not, the time of onset and whether we are dealing with a primary or secondary form. We will also ask about the repercussions on their daily life, impact on sleep, pain that is very annoying or limiting for their social activities (travelling by train, car or plane, not being able to go out for dinner in the evenings, not being able to go to the cinema in the evening or at night, etc.). In any case, the final decision must always be individualised and based on the functional impact of the disease on the patient. It is often useful, in cases of doubt, to carry out a therapeutic attempt so that the patient can judge the benefit he/she would obtain under chronic treatment. In some research studies, an IRLS score of 15 has been used as a scale for deciding when to treat a patient, and this criterion can be used as a benchmark.

If we decide to start a patient with RLS on medication, we must first consider that:

- Drug treatment is symptomatic and does not act on the aetiology of the disease or modify its course. If the medication is stopped, the symptoms usually reappear immediately. Thus, some patients realise that they have forgotten to take their medication when they notice symptoms that had disappeared with treatment.

- The clinical course of RLS is unpredictable. There are subjects in whom RLS only appears for the first time in special situations (during pregnancy, in a state of iron deficiency anaemia, etc.) and then disappears for several years or never reappears in their lifetime. Some patients have a stable chronic course over years or decades; others follow a pattern of flares, with spontaneous remissions and recurrences lasting several months; others experience a progressive worsening of their condition over the years with more intense symptoms, onset at an earlier and earlier time and with a more extensive body localisation, not limited to the legs but encompassing other body areas. Finally, a small group of patients report improvement of RLS over time. It is therefore advisable to periodically attempt to discontinue treatment.

- Some patients present with symptoms only occasionally (less than a day per week) and others very frequently (more than 3 days per week or even daily). In these two forms of presentation, the therapeutic strategy may be different.

- The pathophysiology of RLS is related to defects in the dopaminergic system and iron metabolism and pain control mechanisms. For this reason we can rely on isolated or combined therapeutic strategies to replace the disorders of the dopaminergic system (administering dopaminergic agonists), of iron metabolism (giving iron supplements), or relieving pain (alpha2-delta modulators, opioids), when we wish to initiate pharmacological treatment.

- We must bear in mind that there are secondary forms of RLS, generally associated with iron deficiency and advanced renal failure. In these secondary forms, the initial therapeutic approach may be different from that of the primary form, although it is sometimes necessary to combine symptomatic treatment, similar to that of idiopathic forms, with aetiological treatment. This guideline specifically addresses the treatment of RLS in pregnancy and chronic renal failure.

- We should ask the patient directly if they are taking drugs that may have caused or aggravated RLS, such as antidopaminergics, antidepressants or antihistamines, and see if it is possible to discontinue these treatments.

- We will always recommend proper sleep hygiene, with regular schedules, trying to get the sleep you need and avoiding naps of more than half a night. It is often useful, whenever possible, to delay bedtime, so that the onset of sleep does not coincide with the time of maximum intensity of RLS.

- Non-pharmacological measures (hot or cold water baths, massage, exercise, yoga, relaxation, etc.) may help in some cases to improve symptoms, but are usually not sufficient in moderate and severe cases.

- Our experience in the treatment of RLS is short, as it is only since the late 1990s that articles of acceptable scientific quality began to appear that assessed the efficacy of the drugs. This means that we have a better understanding of drug response in the short term than in the long term in a disease that lasts for years or decades.

- For some medicines we have more scientific information than others because they have received more publications and attention at scientific meetings and conferences. For example, the number of publications and their quality is much higher and better for dopaminergic agents than for opioids and iron supplements. On the other hand, within the same family of medicines, we have more information on some than on others. Thus, for example, among the dopaminergic agents, we have data on the effect of rotigotine at 5 years, but the information we have on the effect of the other dopaminergic agents is less than 2 years. On the other hand, the information we have on alpha2-delta modulators is relatively recent compared to other groups such as dopaminergic agents.

- In Spain, the drugs that "have an indication" at the time of writing (March 2013) are rotigotine, pramipexole and ropinirole. However, other drugs, such as pregabalin or gabapentin enacarbil, already have studies of comparable quality and level of evidence.

- There are effective drugs, such as pergolide, which have been withdrawn from the Spanish market due to serious side effects (cardiac valvular fibrosis). Others, such as gabapentin enacarbil, which have been shown to be effective in various publications, are not yet marketed in Spain at the time of writing.

- If we decide to start a medical treatment, we will do so in monotherapy, in single doses 2-3 hours before the onset of symptoms, at the minimum dose, which we will increase slowly and progressively until symptomatic control is achieved, until the maximum recommended dose is reached or until side effects appear.

- It is essential that the doses used to treat RLS are low, particularly if dopaminergic drugs are used. In general, when symptoms cannot be controlled with 2 mg ropinirole, 0.5 mg pramipexole or 3 mg rotigotine, it is preferable to switch to another drug or to start a combination treatment, for example with an alpha2-delta modulator, rather than to increase the dose further.

- Patients often read the package leaflets of the drugs we have prescribed and may be surprised to read paragraphs about Parkinson's disease and epilepsy. If we prescribe a dopaminergic agent we should tell patients that RLS has no relation to Parkinson's disease. The same goes for epilepsy when prescribing pregabalin.

- We must be prepared for the possibility that in the course of chronic treatment a worsening or tolerance may occur, requiring us to increase the dose, but not to exceed the maximum recommended dose, to add a second drug or to switch to a different drug.

- Drug response is not completely predictable. There are patients who are symptom-free with low doses of a drug and others (although very few) who, with the same baseline symptom intensity, appear to be refractory to all available medications. There are patients who respond very well to one drug family and not to another.

- When a drug is effective, partial or complete improvement of symptoms is usually seen within the first week of treatment. However, the maximum effect is usually seen 2-4 weeks after the start of treatment.

- Special situations may occur. For example, when a patient is going to undergo surgery and their oral RLS medication is to be withdrawn, we can prevent them from becoming unprotected by administering a rotigotine transdermal patch in the days prior to surgery, on the day of surgery and during the postoperative period. We will also advise the patient to advise their surgeon not to administer substituted benzamides such as metoclopramide, and, if antiemetic treatment is required during the operation or in the immediate postoperative period, to use domperidone.

- All drugs that are effective in RLS have side effects. If we decide to give a dopaminergic agent we should warn that it may cause nausea and vomiting, and that in such a case domperidone may be helpful, but that metoclopramide or other benzamides that have an antidopaminergic effect should be avoided. Other possible side effects of dopaminergic drugs are sudden sleep attacks and impulse control disorder. It should be noted that a drug may not be tolerated because of a particular side-effect and another drug of the same pharmacological family and at equivalent doses may not induce this side-effect in a given patient. With rotigotine, the most common side effect is local reactions when administered in the form of a transdermal patch. If cabergoline is administered, it is advisable to perform echocardiograms and chest X-rays every 6 months due to the risk of valvular and pulmonary fibrosis.

- We also have to take into account in daily practice that chronic treatment with dopaminergic agents can be associated with the augmentation phenomenon. This phenomenon is relatively specific to dopaminergic agents. Another aspect to consider, and hardly studied in the medical literature, is that it seems that both dopaminergic and alpha2-delta agents may become tolerant and lose efficacy over time.

8. PHYSIOTHERAPY TREATMENT.

Vertical Push-Ups

Doing vertical bends can help stretch the ligaments, which reduces tension in the legs.

The patient with outstretched arms places the palms of his hands on a wall. Keeping his body straight, he should relax both elbows and bring his chest close to the wall as if doing horizontal push-ups.

Then push the body back slowly to the upright position, not forgetting to keep the palms of both hands flat against the wall. Repeat this movement ten times, and do this exercise twice a day.

Horizontal leg stretches

In this exercise, the patient should lie on their back with one leg raised. Place both hands on the ball of your foot and try to pull your leg over your head. You have to make sure to use only your hands to do this.

This will be slightly painful, but you should hold the position for about three minutes. The effect we are trying to produce is to stretch all the muscles in the back of the leg, making them more flexible and relaxed. Repeat the exercise with the other leg.

Sitting leg stretches

This exercise requires two chairs facing each other and of equal height. The patient should sit on one of the chairs, then lift his leg and put his heel on the seat of the other chair. At this point, the leg should be in a straight line and in front of the patient.

The patient will take a towel and place it on the side of the heel with the foot extended, holding one end of the towel in each of their hands. When he does so, he simply stretches his leg and gently pulls on the towel until he feels his muscles react.

Finally, he/she will carefully lean forward while continuing the tension on the towel. The patient should make sure to keep the back straight. He will hold this position for about thirty seconds, then repeat the process with the other leg. He will perform this exercise twice a day.

A direct interaction between two Restless Legs Syndrome predisposing genes: MEIS1 and SKOR1.

Restless legs syndrome (RLS) is a common sleep disorder for which the genetic contribution remains poorly explained. In 2007, the first genome-wide association study (GWAS) identified three genomic regions associated with RLS. MEIS1, BTBD9 and MAP2K5 / SKOR1 are the only known genes located within these loci and their association with RLS was subsequently confirmed in several follow-up GWAS. Following this finding, our group reported that the MEIS1 risk haplotype is associated with its decreased expression at mRNA and protein levels.

Here we report the effect of risk variants in the other three genes strongly associated with RLS. While these variants had no effect on the mRNA levels of the genes harbouring them, we found that the homeobox transcription factor MEIS1 positively regulates the expression of the transcription co-repressor SKOR1. This regulation is mediated through the binding of MEIS1 at two specific sites located in the promoter region of SKOR1 and is modified by an RLS-associated SNP in the promoter region of the gene.

Our findings directly link MEIS1 and SKOR1, two genes significantly associated with RLS, and also prioritise SKOR1 over MAP2K5 in the RLS-associated intergenic region of MAP2K5 / SKOR1 found by GWAS. (1).

I_h Contributes to increased motor neuron excitability in restless legs syndrome.

Patients with restless legs complain of sensory and motor symptoms that lead to sleep disturbances. Symptoms include painful sensations, urge to move and involuntary leg movements.

The mechanisms responsible for restless legs syndrome are not yet known, but current studies indicate an increased excitability of the neural network. Reflex studies indicate the involvement of spinal structures. Peripheral mechanisms have not been investigated so far.

Here, we provide evidence of increased HCN channel-mediated inward rectification in motor axons. The excitability of sensory axons did not change. We conclude that, in restless legs syndrome, increased HCN current in motor neurons may play a pathophysiological role and that these channels could represent a valuable target for pharmaceutical intervention.

SUMMARY:

Restless legs syndrome is a disorder of the sensorimotor network. So far, the pathophysiological mechanisms responsible are poorly understood. Here, we provide evidence that excitability of peripheral motor neurons contributes to the pathophysiology of restless legs syndrome.

In vivo excitability studies were performed on motor and sensory axons of the median nerve in patients with idiopathic restless legs syndrome (iRLS) who were not currently undergoing treatment. Patients with iRLS had greater adaptation in motor but not sensory axons to long-lasting hyperpolarisation than age-matched healthy subjects, indicating greater inward rectification in iRLS. The most reasonable explanation is that HCN channels open to less hyperpolarised membrane potentials, a view supported by mathematical modelling. The half-activation potential of HCN channels (Bq) [activated by cyclic nucleotide-activated hyperpolarisation] was the best parameter representing the difference between normal controls and iRLS data. A Bq depolarisation of 6 mV reduced the discrepancy between the normal control model and the iRLS data by 92.1%.

Taken together, our results suggest for the first time an increased excitability of motor units in iRLS that could increase the likelihood of leg movements. The abnormal axonal properties are consistent with other findings that the peripheral system is part of the network involved in iRLS (2).

Hyperpolarisation-activated channels activated by cyclic nucleotides potentially modulate axonal excitability at different thresholds.

Hyperpolarisation-activated cyclic nucleotide (HCN)-activated channels mediate differences in sensory and motor axonal excitability at different thresholds in animal models. Importantly, HCN channels are responsible for voltage-gated inward rectifier (Ih) currents activated during hyperpolarisation. Ih currents play a crucial role in determining the resting membrane potential and have been implicated in a variety of neurological disorders, including neuropathic pain.

In humans, differences in the biophysical properties of motor and sensory axons at different thresholds remain to be elucidated and could provide crucial pathophysiological information in peripheral neurological diseases.

Consequently, the aim of this study was to characterise sensory and motor axonal function at different thresholds. Axonal excitability studies of median nerve and sensory axonal excitability were performed in 15 healthy subjects (45 studies in total). Follow-up targets were set at 20, 40 and 60% of maximum for sensory and motor axons. Electrotonic hyperpolarisation threshold (TEh) at 90100 ms was significantly increased in lower-threshold sensory axon thresholds (F = 11.195, P <0.001). In motor axons, the hyperpolarisation current/threshold gradient (I/V) was significantly increased in lower-threshold axons (F = 3.191, P <0.05). The minimum I/V gradient was increased in lower threshold motor and sensory axons.

In conclusion, variation in HCN isoform kinetics could explain the findings in motor and sensory axons. Importantly, assessment of HCN channel function in sensory and motor axons at different thresholds may provide insights into the pathophysiological processes underlying peripheral neurological diseases in humans, with a particular focus on the role of HCN channels with the potential to identify novel treatment targets.

Hyperpolarisation-activated cyclic nucleotide (HCN)-activated channels, which underlie inward rectifier (Ih) currents, appear to mediate differences in sensory and axonal motor properties. Inward rectifier currents increase in lower threshold motor and sensory axons, although different HCN channel isoforms appear to underlie these changes. While faster-activating HCN channels appear to underlie the Ih changes in sensory axons, slower-activating HCN isoforms appear to be mediating the differences in Ih conductances in motor axons of different thresholds.

Differences in the activation properties of HCN could explain the predilection for sensory and motor axon dysfunction in specific neurological diseases (3).

Increased inward canalisation of the HCN channel in fasciculation syndrome with benign cramping

Muscle cramps are a common complaint associated with sudden painful involuntary contractions of a muscle. The mechanisms responsible for muscle cramps are still unclear.

Axonal excitability and multi-unit electromyography studies were performed in 20 patients suffering from fasciculation syndrome with benign cramps, who are currently not taking medication.

Axonal excitability measurements suggested increased inward rectification, indicating an increase in Ih. Mathematical modelling suggested that the data were best explained by depolarisation of the voltage dependence of hyperpolarisation-activated cyclic nucleotide (HCN)-activated channels. Parameters associated with resting membrane potential polarisation were not changed. These findings suggest that a role for HCN channels may manifest during the rhythmic discharge associated with a voluntary contraction. Consistent with this view, patients had higher rates of motor unit discharge than healthy controls during maximal voluntary effort. (4)

Efficacy of vitamin D replacement therapy in restless legs syndrome: a randomised control trial.

PURPOSE:

Restless legs syndrome is a sleep movement disorder that may be related to dopaminergic dysfunction and in which vitamin D may play a role. This 12-week, randomised, placebo-controlled trial elucidated the efficacy of vitamin D supplementation in reducing the severity of restless legs syndrome symptoms.

METHODS:

Thirty-five subjects with restless legs syndrome, diagnosed using the criteria of the International Restless Legs Syndrome Study Group, were enrolled. Subjects were randomised to receive either oral vitamin D (50,000 IU tablets) or placebo. All medications were administered weekly using a direct observation technique. Clinical assessments, including restless legs syndrome severity assessments, were performed at baseline and at the end of the study using the International Restless Legs Syndrome Study Group rating scale. Serum vitamin D levels and bone profiles were measured at baseline and every 4 weeks. The primary endpoint was change in restless legs syndrome severity score from baseline to week 12. There were 17 and 18 patients in the vitamin D and placebo groups, respectively.

RESULTS:

The groups did not differ with respect to age, sex, restless legs syndrome severity or vitamin D levels. Participants in the vitamin D group showed no significant change in mean restless legs syndrome severity score compared to the placebo group.

CONCLUSIONS:

The results suggest that vitamin D supplementation does not improve the symptoms of restless legs syndrome (5).

A study for the mechanism of sensory disturbance in restless legs syndrome based on magnetoencephalography.

Despite the relatively high incidence rate, the aetiology and pathogenesis of restless legs syndrome (RLS) are still unclear. Long-term pharmacological treatments fail to achieve satisfactory curative effects, which is reflected in the rebound and increase of related symptoms.

An electrophysiological endophenotyping experiment was performed to investigate the mechanism of somatosensory disturbance in RLS patients. Together with 15 normal subjects as the control group, with ages and genders comparable to RLS patients, 15 primitive RLS patients were scanned by Magnetoencephalography (MEG) under natural conditions; in addition, the somatosensory evoked magnetic field (SEF) was also measured with single and paired stimuli. Compared to the control group, lower extremity SEF intensities of RLS patients were higher, and paired pulse depression (PPD) for SEF in RLS patients was attenuated. It was also revealed by frequency-time analysis of somatosensory induced oscillation (SIO) in RLS patients that 93.3% of alpha (8-12 Hz) somatosensory induced oscillations were successfully elicited, while 0% gamma (30-55 Hz) somatosensory induced oscillations were elicited; which was significantly different from the control group. Furthermore, in RLS, patients exhibit increased excitability of the sensorimotor cortex, a notable abnormality that exists in early somatosensory activation control (GC) and an attenuated inhibitory interneuron network, which consequently results in a compensatory mechanism through which RLS patients increase their attention. sensory control activation by somatosensory-induced alpha oscillation (8-12 Hz). This hyperexcitability, partly due to electrocortical disinhibition, may have an important therapeutic implication and become an important target for neuromodulatory interventions (6).

Association of mitochondrial iron deficiency and dysfunction with idiopathic restless legs syndrome.

BACKGROUND:

Restless legs syndrome is a sensorimotor neurological disorder of the limbs that affects quality of life and disturbs sleep. However, there have been advances in the understanding of the disease affecting the dopaminergic system as well as iron metabolism. The exact pathophysiological mechanisms of restless legs syndrome remain elusive. We sought to elucidate the mechanisms underlying iron metabolism in subjects with restless legs syndrome at the systemic, cellular and mitochondrial levels.

METHODS:

We conducted a study prospectively recruiting 68 patients with restless legs syndrome and nine age-matched healthy controls that focused on iron metabolism using human monocytes as surrogates.

RESULTS:

Evaluation of parameters of systemic iron metabolism in the circulation showed no significant differences between patients and controls. We observed significantly reduced levels of heme oxygenase 1 mRNA and mitochondrial iron genes such as mitoferrin ly2 in monocytes isolated from patients with restless legs syndrome, indicating mitochondrial iron deficiency. Interestingly, we also observed reduced expression of iron regulatory protein 2 together with altered mitochondrial aconitase activity and reduced mitochondrial superoxide formation in subjects with restless legs syndrome. In this line, patients had reduced mitochondrial respiratory capacity that was improved in restless legs syndrome patients treated with dopaminergic drugs compared to untreated patients.

CONCLUSIONS:

Our data suggest that restless legs syndrome is related to mitochondrial iron deficiency and associated impairment of mitochondrial function. This is partly corrected by treatment with dopaminergic drugs compared to untreated patients, which may be related to an effect of dopamine on cellular iron homeostasis (7).

A prospective, randomised, open-label study comparing the efficacy and safety of Clonazepam versus nortriptyline on quality of life in women over 40 with restless legs syndrome.

Introduction:

Restless legs syndrome (RLS) is a neurological disorder characterised by the urge to move the legs, usually accompanied by unpleasant sensations in the legs. RLS also affects health-related quality of life (QOL) in patients suffering from it. In addition, it affects women more than men. Although a large number of studies are available evaluating the role of benzodiazepines (clonazepam and antidepressant (nortriptyline) in the treatment of RLS, but to our knowledge, there are no comparative studies comparing these two drugs to determine their efficacy and safety). Treatment of RLS QoL among women over 40 years of age.

Materials and methods:

A prospective, randomised, open-label, comparative study was conducted in the postgraduate Department of Pharmacology, in collaboration with the Department of General Medicine, Government Medical College, Jammu, a tertiary teaching hospital for one year.

Conclusion:

Clonazepam proved to be significantly better at improving the RLSQoL score. The difference between the respective baselines of the two groups was statistically insignificant (8).

8.1. Decreased serum ferritin may be associated with increased restless legs syndrome in Parkinson's disease: a meta-analysis for the diagnosis of RLS in patients with PD

Objective:

Restless legs syndrome (RLS) is one of the most common non-motor symptoms of Parkinson's disease (PD), but its pathogenesis in a PD background is unclear. Abnormal iron metabolism may be involved, in which case it may be a risk marker for RLS. Here we conducted a systematic search of the literature and performed a meta-analysis to compare markers of iron metabolism between PD patients with and without RLS.

Method:

PubMed, Embase, Chinese National Knowledge Infrastructure, Wanfang, Web of Science and SinoMed databases were searched for case-control and observational studies examining RLS-related changes in iron metabolism in PD, in terms of serum iron, serum ferritin and haemoglobin. Eligible studies were meta-analyses using Stata 12.0. Results: Meta-analysis of 11 case-control studies showed that serum ferritin concentration was lower in PD patients with RLS than in those without RLS (95% CI -0.32 to -0.03, p=0.018). In contrast, serum iron or haemoglobin levels did not differ significantly between PD patients with or without RLS.

Conclusion:

This meta-analysis may provide the first reliable pooled estimate of the correlation between abnormal iron metabolism and RLS in PD. Available evidence indicates that ferritin levels, but not serum iron or haemoglobin, correlate significantly with RLS in PD, with lower ferritin levels correlating with a higher prevalence of RLS(9).

Association between restless legs syndrome symptoms and self-reported hypertension: a nationwide questionnaire study in Korea.

Background

The association between restless legs syndrome (RLS) and hypertension remains controversial. We investigated the relationship between RLS and hypertension in a national sample of the Korean adult population.

METHODS:

This was a cross-sectional questionnaire-based study involving 2,740 adults aged 19 years and older. Subjects who met the four essential criteria of the International RLS Study Group and reported symptoms occurring at least once a week were defined as the RLS group. The presence of hypertension was defined as a self-reported history of hypertension diagnosed by a physician. Multiple logistic regression analysis was performed to determine the independent association between RLS symptoms and self-reported hypertension after adjusting for potential confounders.

RESULTS:

Among the 2,740 subjects, 68 (2.5%; 95% confidence interval [CI], 1.9% -3.1%) had RLS with a symptom frequency of at least once a week. The prevalence of self-reported hypertension was 30.9% (95% CI, 20.5% -42.0%) in the RLS group, which was significantly higher than in controls (12.4%; 95% CI, 11.2% -13.6%; P < 0.001). Multiple logistic regression analysis showed that the adjusted odds ratio for self-reported hypertension in the RLS group was 2.10 (95% CI, 1.12-3.93) compared with controls. In addition to RLS symptoms, older age, overweight, low education level, diabetes mellitus and short sleep duration were significantly associated with self-reported hypertension.

CONCLUSION:

RLS symptoms occurring at least once a week are independently associated with a higher prevalence of self-reported hypertension in the Korean adult population. Further research will confirm the clinical implication of the current findings and the causal relationship between RLS and hypertension.(lO).

Impact of different stages of chronic kidney disease on the severity of Willis-Ekbom disease.

Introduction

Willis-Ekbom syndrome (WED) / restless legs syndrome (RLS) is a disorder in which the patient has neurological features, such as the need for rhythmic limb movement, which may slow down or stop when the limb is moved. In this study, we sought to compare the severity of WED at different stages of chronic kidney disease (CKD).

Materials and methods:

In this study, a total of 300 patients with CKD who were over 18 years of age were included. All participants underwent a questionnaire for the diagnosis of RLS (essential clinical criteria for the diagnosis of RLS) and a questionnaire on the International Restless Legs Syndrome Study Group Rating Scale for severity.

Observation and results:

Our study showed a 20% prevalence of WED in CKD patients. CKD patients on haemodialysis had significantly more WED than the conservative group (P = 0.0001). Patients with a history of diabetes mellitus showed a significant correlation with WED (P = 0.026), while patients with a history of hypertension showed both diabetes mellitus and hypertension and smoking had no significant relationship with WED (P = 0.27, P = 0.23, and P = 0.22, respectively). The different stages of CKD showed a significant correlation with WED (P = 0.002), with more WED among CKD patients in stage V. WED was more in haemodialysis patients (P = 0.0001). The correlation of different stages of CKD with severity of WED was statistically significant (P = 0.029), with WED being more severe among stage V CKD.

Conclusion:

WED was more frequent among CKD patients on maintenance haemodialysis and diabetes mellitus. However, no such relationship could be established for hypertension alone. Patients with higher grades of CKD were more likely to have symptoms of WED, and the severity of these symptoms increases with the stages of CKD(ll).
Serum C-reactive protein / albumin ratio and restless legs syndrome.

OBJECTIVES:

Our study aimed to assess the variation in serum C-reactive protein/albumin (CAR) ratio, a biomarker of peripheral inflammation and oxidative stress, in patients with restless legs syndrome (RLS).

METHODS:

The study included a total of 380 individuals, including 197 with a diagnosis of RLS. The diagnosis of RLS was determined according to the "International Restless Legs Syndrome Study Group" questionnaire. Disease severity was assessed according to the "International Restless Legs Syndrome Study Group Severity Scale".

RESULTS:

The mean age of the restless legs syndrome patients was 52.5 ± 12.7 years, while the mean age in the control group was 50.8 ± 11.2, with no statistically significant differences (p = 0.156). Haemoglobin, iron and ferritin levels in the patient group were lower than in the control group (p<0.001; p<0.01; p<0.001), with total iron binding capacity levels higher than the control group (p<0.001). Mean ferritin in the RLS group (49.8 ± 51.2) was lower than the control group (76.9 ± 44.7). In patients, the ratio of C-reactive protein, albumin and C-reactive protein/albumin was found to be 0.21 ± 0.18, 4.43 ± 0.31 and 0.07 ± 0.05, respectively. When compared to the control group, the patient group had high C-reactive protein (CRP), CAR and low albumin levels (p<0.001). Among patients with "very severe" disease severity, ferritin levels were found to be lower than those with "moderate" disease severity. In addition, patients with "very severe" disease had albumin levels that were significantly lower compared to those with "mild" disease severity (p<0.05).

CONCLUSION:

Our study supports the hypothesis that serum albumin, ferritin, CRP and CAR levels may be associated with restless legs syndrome(12).

Association between serum hepcidin level and restless legs syndrome.

BACKGROUND:

To better understand the role of dysregulation of iron homeostasis in restless legs syndrome, we compared serum hepcidin and ferritin levels in drug-naïve patients with primary restless legs syndrome and healthy controls, and studied the relationship between hepcidin level and severity of restless legs syndrome.

METHODS:

One hundred and eight drug-free patients with primary restless legs syndrome (65 women; mean age, 61.5 years) and 45 controls (28 women; mean age, 53.9 years) were included. Inclusion criteria were: normal ferritin level (> 50 ng/ml) and absence of iron disorders, chronic renal or hepatic insufficiency and inflammatory or neurological diseases. Each subject underwent a complete clinical examination and polysomnography evaluation. Serum hepcidin-25 was quantified using a validated mass spectrometry method. The severity of restless legs syndrome was assessed according to the International Restless Legs Syndrome Study Group.

RESULTS:

Although there was no group difference between normal ferritin levels and demographic characteristics, serum hepcidin level and hepcidin/ferritin ratio were higher in patients than in controls. Hepcidin level and hepcidin/ferritin ratio, but not ferritin level, were positively correlated with periodic leg movements during sleep and wakefulness in the whole sample. Hepcidin level appears to be associated with restless legs syndrome severity in a complex U-shaped relationship, unrelated to age at onset of restless legs syndrome, positive family history, sleep and depressive symptoms, genetic background and polysomnographic measurements. No relationship was found between ferritin level and severity of restless legs syndrome.

CONCLUSION:

In drug-naïve patients with primary restless legs syndrome, the hepcidin level is higher than in controls and may be associated with the clinical severity of restless legs syndrome. This result emphasises the complex dysregulation of peripheral iron metabolism in restless legs syndrome, opening up potential prospects for a personalised approach with a hepcidin antagonist (13).

Relationship of the International Restless Legs Syndrome Study Group rating scale with the Clinical Global Impression severity scale, the 6-item Restless Legs Syndrome Questionnaire and the Restless Legs Syndrome Quality of Life Questionnaire.

BACKGROUND:

The SP790 study (ClinicalTrials.gov, NCT00136045) showed the benefits of rotigotine over placebo in improving the severity of symptoms of restless legs syndrome

(RLS), also known as Willis-Ekbom disease, on the International Restless Legs Syndrome Study Group (IRLS) Clinical Global Impression Item 1 (CGI-1) rating scale, the 6-item RLS questionnaire (RLS-6) and the RLS Quality of Life Questionnaire (RLS-QoL) in patients with moderate to severe idiopathic RLS. To provide a clinical context for the IRLS and to guide the choice of assessment scales for RLS studies, our post hoc analysis of SP790 data assessed the associations between the IRLS and CGI-1, the IRLS and RLS-6, and the IRLS and RLS-QoL .

METHODS:

Scale associations were analysed at baseline and end-of-maintenance (EoM) using data from the safety set (rotigotine and placebo groups combined [n=458]). Changes from baseline to EoM in IRLS score versus comparator scale scores were also analysed.

RESULTS:

There was a tendency for the IRLS severity category to increase with increasing CGI-1, RLS-6 and RLS-QoL. Pearson product moment correlation coefficients showed correlations between IRLS and comparison scale scores at baseline and MoU, as well as correlations for change from baseline to MoU.

CONCLUSION:

The correlations between the IRLS and the comparative scales were substantial. These data indicate that the IRLS is clinically meaningful. The IRLS and CGI-1 are generally sufficient to assess the overall severity and impact of RLS symptoms in clinical trials (14).

The short-term effects of olive oil massage on the severity of uremic restless legs syndrome: a double-blind, placebo-controlled trial.

BACKGROUND:

Although the efficacy of olive oil massage has been established for different disorders, no study has yet focused on the effect of olive oil massage on restless legs syndrome (RLS). In this study, we aimed to evaluate the short-term effects of olive oil massage in reducing the severity of uraemic RLS.

METHODS:

This double-blind, placebo-controlled trial was conducted in 60 patients with uraemic RLS (mean age: 51.96 ± 10.15), who were randomly divided into olive oil and placebo groups. The olive oil group received an olive oil massage, while the placebo group received a liquid paraffin massage twice a week during haemodialysis sessions for three weeks. For each leg, 10 ml of olive oil or placebo was applied and then massaged for five minutes from the plantar surface of the foot to the area below the knee. The severity of RLS was assessed on the first day and one week after the final massage therapy session using the International Restless Legs Syndrome Study Group Rating Scale (IRLSSG).

RESULTS:

In terms of different categories of RLS severity, a significant decrease was observed only in the olive oil group from pre- to post-intervention stages ($P = 0.003$). After the intervention, the decrease in total RLS severity was more significant in the olive oil group ($P < 0.001$) compared to the placebo group ($P = 0.019$). In addition, a significant difference in total RLS severity ($P < 0.001$) and different categories of RLS severity ($P = 0.002$) was observed after the intervention between the groups in favour of olive oil massage. However, no significant differences were found between the groups at the pre-intervention stage in this regard ($P = 0.363$ and $P = 0.955$, respectively).

CONCLUSION:

Short-term application of olive oil massage as an adjunctive method appears to be effective in reducing the severity of uraemic RLS. Further studies are suggested to identify the sustainability of the findings(15).

Impact of different stages of chronic kidney disease on the severity of Willis-Ekbom disease.

Introduction:

Willis-Ekbom syndrome (WED) / restless legs syndrome (RLS) is a disorder in which the patient has neurological features, such as the need for rhythmic limb movement, which may slow down or stop when the limb is moved. In this study, we sought to compare the severity of WED at different stages of chronic kidney disease (CKD).

Materials and methods:

In this study, a total of 300 patients with CKD who were over 18 years of age were included. All participants underwent a questionnaire for the diagnosis of RLS (essential clinical criteria for the diagnosis of RLS) and a questionnaire on the International Restless Legs Syndrome Study Group Rating Scale for severity.

Observation and results:

Our study showed a 20% prevalence of WED in CKD patients. CKD patients on haemodialysis had significantly more WED than the conservative group (P = 0.0001). Patients with a history of diabetes mellitus showed a significant correlation with WED (P = 0.026), while patients with a history of hypertension showed both diabetes mellitus and hypertension and smoking had no significant relationship with WED (P = 0.27, P = 0.23, and P = 0.22, respectively). The different stages of CKD showed a significant correlation with WED (P = 0.002), with more WED among CKD patients in stage V. WED was more in haemodialysis patients (P = 0.0001). The correlation of different stages of CKD with severity of WED was statistically significant (P = 0.029), with WED being more severe among stage V CKD.

Conclusion:

WED was more frequent among CKD patients on maintenance haemodialysis and diabetes mellitus. However, no such relationship could be established for hypertension alone. Patients with higher grades of CKD were more likely to have symptoms of WED, and the severity of these symptoms increases with the stages of CKD(16).

Brain iron accumulation in a family of blood donors with restless legs syndrome.

INTRODUCTION:

The pathophysiology of restless legs syndrome (RLS) is complex. Secondary RLS with iron deficiency, suggesting a disturbance of iron homeostasis, remains to be elucidated.

CASE REPORTS:

We present findings from a single blood donor family with RLS. Three blood donor relatives were diagnosed with RLS as defined by the International RLS Study Group and with no history of neurological diseases and symptoms of RLS in the last 3-5 years (blood donation range: 10-40 years). Neurological examination and electromyography were normal. A polysomnography showed disturbed nocturnal sleep with reduced sleep efficiency and increased rate of periodic limb movement. Cranial magnetic resonance imaging showed iron deposits in the brain in the basal ganglia, substantia nigra, red nuclei and dentate nuclei. Phenotypic and genotypic studies ruled out genetic haemochromatosis or iron overload.

CONCLUSION:

The abnormal accumulation of iron in the basal ganglia indicated a complex disorder of iron metabolism in the central nervous system. Further studies are required to confirm our findings and their role in the pathophysiology of RLS (17).

Extracellular vesicles reveal abnormalities in neuronal iron metabolism in restless legs syndrome.

Aims of the study To determine abnormalities in the levels of iron control proteins in neuronal enriched extracellular vesicles (nEV) in restless legs syndrome (RLS).

METHODS:

We used immunoprecipitation for the neuronal marker L1CAM to isolate nEVs from the serum of 20 RLS subjects from a study that included MRI determinations of substantia nigra iron deposition and haematological parameters and 28 age- and sex-matched controls.

RESULTS:

RLS compared to control subjects showed higher levels of total ferritin nEV but similar levels of transferrin receptor and ferroportin. Western transfer analysis showed that heavy chain but not light chain ferritin was increased in RLS nEV compared to control subjects. In RLS but not Control subjects, nEV total ferritin correlated positively with systemic iron parameters; the two groups also differed in the ratio of nEV total ferritin to MRI measures of iron deposition in the substantia nigra.

CONCLUSIONS:

Given the neuronal origin and diversity of EV load, nEVs provide an important platform for exploring the underlying pathophysiology and potential biomarkers of RLS.(18).

Restless Legs Syndrome is a disorder of the sensorimotor network. Recent studies have shown that increased HCN current in motor neurons may trigger a pathophysiological role underlying peripheral neurological diseases in humans.

This finding may provide new treatments for a disorder with an as yet unclear pathogenesis. What does seem to be increasingly clear is that abnormal iron metabolism may be involved, with lower ferretin levels occurring. RLS is also associated with a higher prevalence of self-reported hypertension, although there is controversy between studies.

BIBLIOGRAPHY.

Catoire h, Sarayloo F, Mourabit Amarik, Apuzzo S, Grant A, Rochefort D, Xiong L...et al. A direct interaction between two Restless Legs Syndrome predisposing genes: MEIS1 and SKOR1. Sci Rep 2018 Aug 15 ;(!): 12173. doi: 10.1038/s41598-018-30665-6.

1. Czesnik D, Howells J, Bartl M, Veiz E, Ketzer R, Kemmet O, Walters AS...et al. .et al. Ih contributes to increased motoneuron excitability in restless legs syndrome. J Physiol. 2018Nov 14. doi: 10.1113/JP275341.

2. Weerasinghe D, Menon P 6 Vocics. Hyperpolarization-activated cyclic-ucleotide-gated channels potentially modulate axonal excitability at different thresholds. J Neurophysiol. 2017 Dec 1;   118(6):3044-3050. doi: 10.1152/jn.00576.2017. Epub 2017 Sep 13

3. Czesnik D, Howells J, Negrof, Wagenknecht M, Hanner S, Farina D, Burke D..et al. Increased HCN channel driven inward rectification in benign cramp fasciculation syndrome. Brain 2015 Nov; 138 (Pt11): 3168-79. Doi: 10.1093/brain/awv254. Epub 2015 Sep 5.

4. Walim SO, Abaalkhail B, Alhejaili F & Pandi-Perumal SR. Efficacy of vitamin D replacement therapy in restless legs syndrome: a randomized control trial. Sleep Breath. 2018 Nov 14. Doi. 10.1007/s 11325-018-1751-2.

5. Yang H, Wang L, li X, Wang K, Hou Y, Zhang X, Chen Z...et al. A study for the mechanism of sensory disorder in restless legs syndrome based on magnetoencephalography. Sleep Med. 2018 Sep 22; 53: 35-44. Doi: 10.1016/ j.sleep.2018.07.026.

6. Haschka D, Volani C, Stefani A, Tymoszuk P, Mitterling T, Holzknecht E, Heidbreder A...et al. Association of mitochondrial iron deficiency and dysfunction with idiopathic restless legs syndrome. Mov Disord 2018 Oct 11. Doi: 10.1002/mds.27482.

7. Roshi,Tandon VR, Mahajan A, Sharma S, Khajuria V. A Prospective, Randomized, Open-Label Study Comparing the Efficacy and Safety of

Clonazepam versus Nortriptyline on Quality of Life in 40+ Years oíd Women Presenting with Restless Leg Syndrome. J Midlife Health.2018 Jul-Sep; 9(3): 135-139. Doi: 10.4103/jmh.JMH_25_18.

8. Kelu Li, Bin Liu, Fang Wang, Jianjian Bao, Chungmin Wu, Xiaodong Huang, Fatun Hu..et al.Decreased Serum ferritin may be associated with increased restless legs syndrome in P/rkinson's disease: a meta-analysis for the diagnosis of RLS in PD patients.Int j Neurosci. 2019 May 16:1-11. doi: 10.1080/00207454.2019.1608200.

9. Sunwoo JS, Kim WJ, Chu MK & Yang KI.Association between Restless Legs Syndrome Symptoms and Self-Reported Hypertension: a Nationwide Questionnaire Study in Korea. J Korean Med Sci. 2019 Apr 29; 34 (16): e130. Doi: 10.3346/jkms.2019.34.e130.

10. Bhagawati J, Kumar S, Agrawal AK, Acharya S, Wanjari AK & Kamble TK.Impact of different stages of chronic kidney disease on the severity of Willis-Ekbom disease. J Family Med Prim Care. 2019 Feb;8 (2): 432-436. Doi:10.4103/jfmpc.jfmpc_418_18.

11. Olgun Yazar H, Yazar T, Ozdemir S & Kasko Arici Y. Serum C-reactive protein / albumin ratio and retless legs syndrome. Sleep Med. 2019 Mar 14;58:61-65. doi: 10.1016/j.sleep.2019.02.022.

12. Dauvilliers Y, Chenini S, Vialaret J, Delaby C, Guiraud L, Gaballe A, Lopez R...et al. Association between serum hepcidin level and restless syndome. Mov Disord. 2018 apr,33(4):618-627. Doi: 10.1002/mds.27287.

13. Allen R, Oertel W, Walters A, Benes H, Schollmayer E, Grieger F, Moran K...et al. Relation of the international restless Legs Syndrome Study Group rating scale with the Clinical Global Impression severity scalke, the restless legs syndrome 6-item questionnaire, and the restless legs syndrome-quality of life questionnaire. Sleep Med 2013Dec ;14(12):1375-80. Doi: 10.1016/j.sleep.2013.09.008.

14. Nasiri m, Abbasi M, Khosroabadi ZY, Sagafi H, Hamzeei F, Amiri MH & Yusefi

H. Short-term effects of massage with olive oil on the severity of uremic restlessness.

legs syndrome: A double-blind placebo-controlled trial. Complement Ther Med. 2019 Jun; 44:261-268. doi: 10.1016/j.ctim.2019.05.009.

15. Bhagawati J, Kumar S, Agrawal AK, Acharya S, Wanjari AK & Kamble TK. Impact of different stages of chronic kidney disease on the severity of Willis-Ekbom disease. J Family Med Prim Care. 2019 Feb;8(2):432-436. Doi: 10.4103/jfmpc.jfmpc_418_18.

16. Lillo-Triguero L, Del Castillo A, Guzman de Villoría J, Moran-Jimenez MJ, Guillem A & Peraita- Adrados R. Brain iron accumulation in a blood donor family with resless legs syndrome. Rev Neural. 2019 Feb 1;68(3):107-110.

17. Chawla S, Gulyani S, Allen RP, Earley CJ, Li X, Van Zijil P & Kapogiannis D. Extracellular Vesicles Reveal Abnormalities In Neuronal Iron Metabolism In Restless Legs Syndrome Sleep. 2019 Mar 21. pii: zsz079. Doi: 10.1093/sleep/zsz079.

Table of contents

1. INTRODUCTION 1
2. DEFINITION 2
3. EPIDEMIOLOGY 5
4. AETIOLOGY AND PATHOPHYSIOLOGY 6
5. CLINICAL PICTURE AND SPECIFIC SCALES FOR THE ASSESSMENT OF SYMPTOM SEVERITY 12
6.DIAGNOSIS 16
7. TREATMENT. 17
8. PHYSIOTHERAPY TREATMENT. 22
9. RESEARCH ARTICLES 23
CONCLUSION. 41
BIBLIOGRAPHY 42

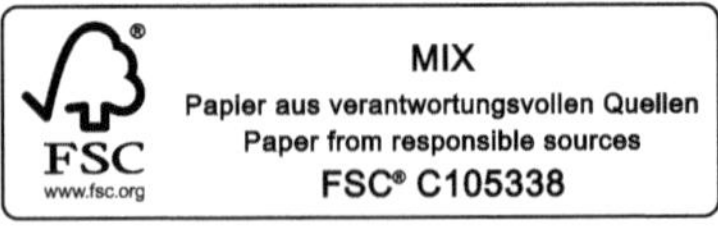

Printed by Books on Demand GmbH, Norderstedt / Germany